Understanding
Indian Head
Massage

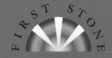

F I R S T   S T O N E

Contents

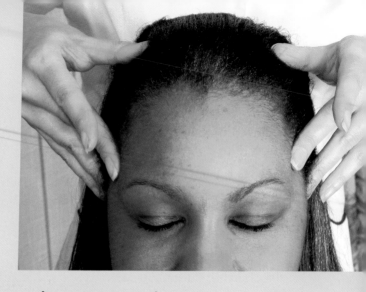

1

Understanding
Indian Head Massage

Indian head massage is growing fast in popularity and has been hailed as the therapy of the 21st century.

It is based on an ancient Eastern form of healing, which relaxes and harmonises the body's natural balance, in turn promoting physical, psychological and emotional well-being.

Indian head massage, properly applied, reduces muscular and nervous tension, and improves circulation. The improved circulation helps to detoxify the body, leaving a feeling of tranquillity and inner calm.

> *The improved circulation helps to detoxify the body*

The therapy is carried out in a seated position. It is usual for soothing music to accompany the massage, promoting relaxation in the client.

During a treatment, the client places both feet on the floor with their eyes closed. Treatment should begin with a few deep breaths.

In most cases, the therapist speaks to the client only if there is any discomfort or a problem.

Indian head massage is carried out over clothing and covers the following areas:

- **Upper back/arms:** The upper back is worked on using techniques that should promote relaxation, at the same time releasing knotted tension from the trapezius muscle.
- **Neck:** A slightly gentler approach is taken in this area, which is generally prone to hold the type of tension that causes stiffness and aching.
- **Scalp:** As well as releasing tension from the muscles, we must also consider tension that is held in the bones.

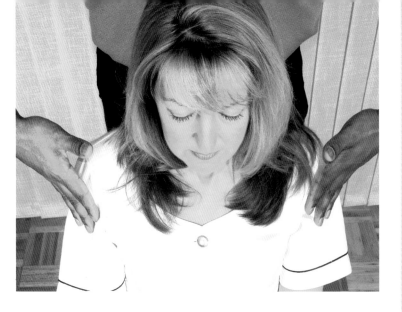

Here the practitioner is working on the upper back and arms, finishing the flow from the back before beginning on the neck. This will relieve shoulder tension.

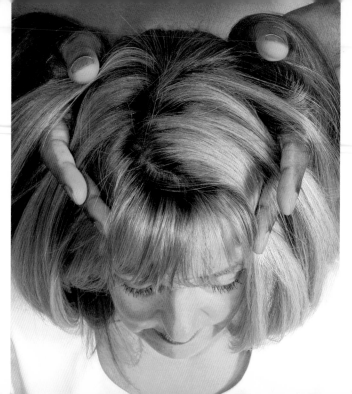

Applying Indian head massage to the scalp helps to relieve tension and stress.

- **Face/ears:** A gentler approach is used here when finishing off the massage. The client is left feeling relaxed and balanced.

The techniques used are designed to relax and stimulate, and there should be no sudden, sharp moves by the therapist. At no time should the client feel uncomfortable or uneasy.

As an alternative, an oil scalp massage can be administered. This is an invigorating, stimulating massage, which promotes increased circulation in the blood vessels of the scalp.

COMMUNICATION THROUGH TOUCH

It has been said that only seven per cent of all communication is verbal. This says a lot for the ability to communicate via the power of touch.

The power of touch is generally better understood in the cultures of the East than it is in the West. In India, home of head massage, communication through touching is a part of everyday life.

This tactile lifestyle conveys a sense of belonging and acts as a tool for communicating what words cannot say. Through massage we are able to help those who are not used to conveying feelings through the power of touch. It can be quite a revelation to some recipients!

For instance, Indian head massage is used successfully on patients in hospices, the aged and infirm – those whose lives are made easier through a sense of closeness and comfort.

By using the power of touch, the therapist is able to communicate compassion and deep empathy. The therapist's hands are used skilfully to massage the back, neck, scalp, face and ears, using techniques that, although they are applied on the body's surface, act deeply within the recipient.

Communication by touch is a powerful tool and a vital part of authentic Indian head massage. The therapist must practise his or her art with

The power of touch –
communicating
through the hands –
is an essential tool
for the Indian head
massage therapist.

compassion, otherwise we are delivering mere mechanical movements that have little lasting effect.

Applying harsh touch can even be counter-productive, causing the body to defend itself and rendering the technique ineffective. Aggressive massage can cause mental, physical, and sometimes emotional distress.

With effective, gentle touch we are stimulating the nervous system and promoting mental, social and physical development. This healthy communication leads to a sense of comfort and compassion.

So the aim of the therapist is to use physical touch to convey a sense of companionship, comfort and communication.

AYURVEDA

Head massage is a therapy that has developed from Eastern ayurvedic medicine and massage. The word ayurveda is made up of two words from one of the oldest languages known to man: Sanskrit.

Ayur means 'life' and *veda* means 'knowledge'. Combined as ayurveda, the word signifies the 'science of life'. Ayurveda is one of the oldest forms of medicine in the world, originating in India more than 2,500 years ago.

There are several basic principles to ayurveda. They and are as follows:

- Ayurveda follows a science based on man's environment and it has been developed through Indian philosophy and culture.
- It has a universal approach that can be applied throughout the world.
- It is based on the scientific principles of diagnostics, pathology, pharmacology and physiology.
- The ayurvedic approach is also an holistic one, encompassing the whole person, mentally, physically and emotionally. This is sometimes referred to as body, soul and spirit.
- Ayurveda states that there are three elementary functional principles that maintain equilibrium in the

body. These are called the three doshas: Kapha, Pitta and Vayu.

- Ayurvedic medicine uses vegetables, metals, animal products, gems and semi-precious stones.
- Ayurvedic therapy concentrates on the person rather than the disease. Each person's constitution is different.
- Ayurveda is an 'environmentally friendly' therapy that holds that we are part of nature and nature is part of us.

BALANCING THE CHAKRAS

One of the most important principles behind the techniques applied in Indian head massage concerns balancing those vital elements known as the body's energy chakras.

Chakras are spinning wheels of energy linked to our various systems. They work on the psychological, physical and emotional parts of a human being.

The ayurvedic element in head massage means that the

therapist works on the following chakras:

- Crown chakra
- Throat chakra
- Heart chakra

By successfully combining skilled touch with ayurvedic knowledge, the Indian head massage therapist can rebalance the chakras and so promote physical, psychological and emotional well-being.

See pages pages 16-17 for more information on the various chakras.

FURTHER APPLICATIONS

The therapy, despite its name, is not just for the head. When properly applied, authentic Indian head massage acts as a de-stressing programme for the whole body.

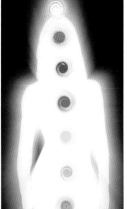

The skilled practitioner is able to to promote a subtle healing energy in the body.

THE CHAKRAS

Chakra	Eastern name	Physical attributes	Representation
Crown	Sahasrara	Brain, pineal gland	Relating to universal energies
Third eye	Ajna	Forehead, lower brain, pituitary gland, nervous system	Relating to psychic and intuitive awareness
Throat	Vishudha	Vocal system	Relating to speech and sound
Heart	Anahata	Heart, thymus and circulatory system	Relating to the soul and emotions
Solar plexus	Manipura	Stomach, diaphragm, nervous system, and liver	Relating to spirituality – connection to universal and earthly energies
Sacral	Svadhistana	Reproductive system	Relating to the beginning of physical life
Base	Muladhara	Perinuem	Foundation of the physical

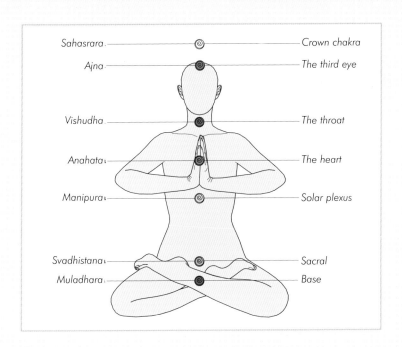

Sahasrara — Crown chakra

Ajna — The third eye

Vishudha — The throat

Anahata — The heart

Manipura — Solar plexus

Svadhistana — Sacral

Muladhara — Base

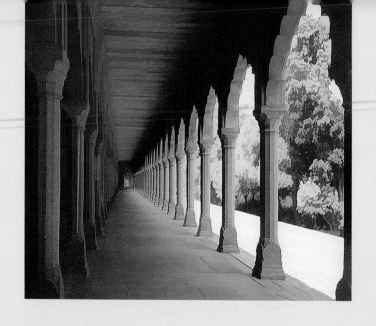

2

East Meets West

Centuries ago Indian head massage was developed as part of a family "grooming tradition" in Indian households.

It later developed as a treatment and was offered by barbers and ayurvedic practitioners or therapists.

The skills of Indian head massage have been handed down through generations, and, in the past, were often linked to a family trade.

Within the home, head massage was developed by family members, who used various oils according to the season. It was also used as a treatment for the hair.

The skills of head massage were passed down through generations

The use of oils was a way of keeping the hair strong, healthy and lustrous. Oils such as coconut, sesame seed, mustard and sweet almond would be used according to the time of year and mental attitude of the recipient. The use of oils would stimulate and refresh the individual, as well as provide a sense of well-being.

Head massage has always played an important role in India as an holistic healing method. Many babies would receive daily massage, up to the age of six years. Later on, the children would begin to massage other members of the family. Head massage runs across the generations as an integral part of family life.

Today you can receive a variation on the original head massage as part of a grooming process. It can be found in many different areas of India, from barbers' shops to markets – even on the beaches.

In the last 30 years a variation on Indian head massage has developed that

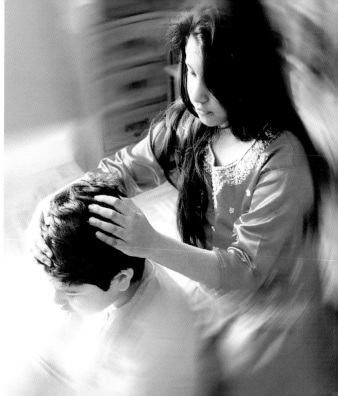

In many traditional Indian homes, children learn the skills of head massage and apply them to their younger brothers and sisters.

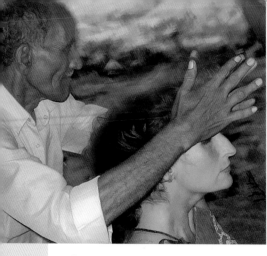

In India, you will often see Indian head massge being given on the beach.

brings into play different areas of the body – the back, neck, face, arms and ears. All of these areas are vulnerable and can hold much stress and tension. By applying different degrees of pressure, a rhythmic massage is applied, which releases various stresses.

EAST MEETS WEST

When looking at Indian head massage it is very important to understand that there are several reasons why an adaptation of the traditional massage, as applied in its native country, is necessary.

THE CLIMATE

It has been claimed that, in India, climate influences the strength of the body's skeleton.

The action of the hot sun promotes greater strength in the bones, allowing a strong massage. Indian head massage applied in the East is more of a vigorous massage and suits the clients there; their skeletal and muscular system is built for the treatment. A similar massage carried out in a cold climate would cause problems for those who did not have such strong bones.

It is always wise to explain your tolerance level of pressure to the therapist, so the massage does not cause any pain.

POSITIVE MENTAL ATTITUDE

The general attitude of the

East is driven by fate, culture, religion and a belief that things are better out than in!

In the West we are more conservative and repressive, harbouring stress and tension in our bodies. This can cause us many problems mentally, physically and emotionally as life goes by.

DIET

The Indian diet is very much built around fresh fruit and vegetables, which help to detoxify the body and promote well-being.

After all, we are what we eat! In the West we tend to rely heavily on processed and pre-prepared foods with many additives and preservatives – fast foods and snacks are big culprits.

These additives tend to affect the body, causing imbalances that eventually have to be resolved if good physical (as well as mental and spiritual) health is to prevail.

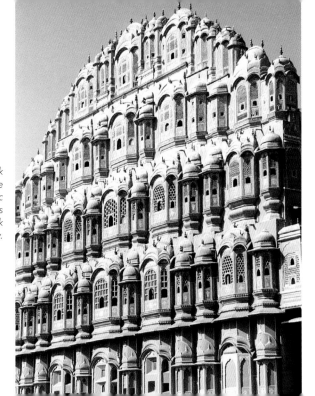

The Pink Palace, where Ayurdevic practitioners would work for royalty.

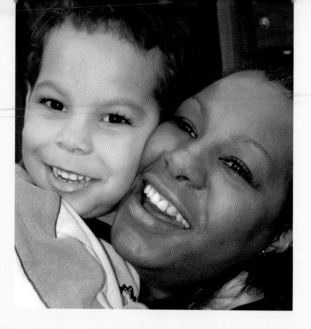

3

Stress Management

Stress is one of the most dangerous afflictions known to man and can attack at any time. It is unmistakable in experience, yet is easier seen in others than in oneself!

Stress is one of the main roots of bad health on all three levels: mental, physical and emotional.

IDENTIFYING STRESS
Today this 'disease' is better understood in the West. Significant measure are being taken to help people help themselves against this scourge of modern society, this potential killer.

The four aspects of your life that need attention when dealing with stress are as follows:
• Work
• Health
• Lifestyle
• Relationships.

Stress can and does affect all of the above. This means that, in order to combat stress, stress management needs to become part of your daily life.

Stress itself is not always a bad thing; it is only a problem if it builds to excessive levels over a long period of time.

A certain amount of pressure can lead to greater achievements, resulting in more self-confidence, e.g. if one wants to excel in sport, a certain amount of stress is necessary to provide the motivation to perform and compete.

Positive stress prepares you for action and provides motivation to cope with everyday life: everything from achieving goals and ambitions to coping with (and getting the most out of) such events as a family wedding.

What determines whether a particular situation is stressful or not is determined by the balance of external demands, internal needs and values, personal coping, resources and external support.

The body's response to stress prepares it for fight or flight; today's lifestyles do not usually allow us to do either, so the body is left in a tense and alert state.

SYMPTOMS OF STRESS

Physical
(Effect on the body)

- Headache or migraine
- Indigestion
- Raised blood pressure
- Neck or backache
- Muscle tension
- Addiction to medication or drugs
- Impotence
- Constipation
- Irritable bowel syndrome

Psychological
(Effect on the mind)

- Mental tiredness
- Anxiety
- Anger
- Phobias
- Poor concentration
- Depression
- Low self-esteem
- Feelings of hopelessness
- Irritability
- Excessive tearfulness

Excessive stress is very harmful, leading to heart, respiratory and digestive disorders, muscle tension, allergies, accidents and mental illness.

HEADACHE

One of the most common stress-related complaints is headache. One in three individuals consult their doctor with this symptom every year, and 95 per cent of the population suffers from headaches at some time.

Massaging the scalp, face, neck, ears and shoulders relieves headaches and eyestrain, improves concentration, eliminates muscle tension, and helps joint mobility.

Massage also eliminates muscle tension and restores joint movement by stretching and mobilising the tissues of the neck and shoulders.

GENERAL HEALTH

The immune system also receives a boost, and a general feeling of well-being is created. Indian head massage attacks

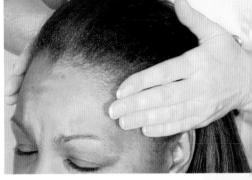

Indian head massage is an ideal way of managing stress.

stress in an immediate way by bringing instant beneficial physical effects. It also aids better relaxation and sleep, the lack of which is often a strong component in stress-related illnesses that can lead to more serious mental breakdown.

STRESS MANAGEMENT

Using a therapy such as Indian head massage is a great way of managing stress. It has been proven to be a very successful method of balancing the mental, emotional and physical aspects of the individual.

Someone thus balanced finds it easier to work through a rational thought process, so he or she is able to manage his or her own stress levels.

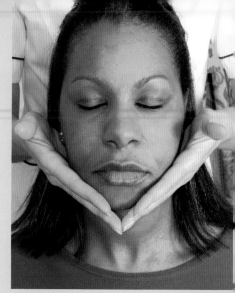

4

How
Head
Massage
Can
Work
For You

Indian head massage has become increasingly popular in the West, and more and more therapists are choosing to add it to their lists of treatments available.

Examining boards now run courses in Indian head massage across Britain. It is currently the fastest growing therapy and is offered as a standard treatment in many health centres, clinics, beauty establishments, hospitals, hospices and doctors' surgeries.

Training in the application of Indian head massage should provide a comprehensive

Head massage is currently the fastest growing therapy in the West

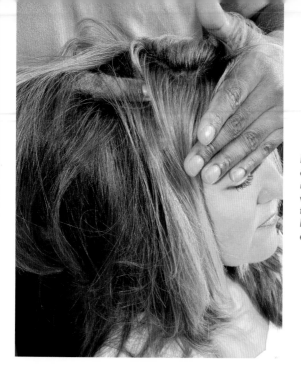

Deep penetration of the scalp releases stress, and will help the client to manage stress in his or her life more effectively.

grounding in the theoretical basis and practical application, so that therapists can implement the technique within their professional practice.

The purpose behind the treatment is to improve the client's ability to cope with stress levels and encourage a more holistic approach to their lives.

Regular home-care or after-care is essential. Appropriate exercise to suit the client's individual needs should be encouraged.

THE BENEFITS OF INDIAN HEAD MASSAGE

The benefits of the head massage are physical, psychological and emotional. A few common physical benefits are as follows:

- It creates a general relaxation of the muscles, as well as speeding up the rate of toxic elimination through better working of the lymphatic drainage system
- It stimulates the flow of blood to the areas massaged, increasing the levels of oxygen in those

tissues particularly important to brain function
- It relieves symptoms of congestion, insomnia, eye strain and tinnitus.

This is not an exhaustive list and further benefits have been widely noted by practitioners.

Clients treated with Indian head massage have recorded the following psychological and emotional benefits:
- A sense of tranquillity
- Improvements in alertness
- Increased mental focus and vision
- A feeling of well-being
- An inner calmness
- An empowered feeling.

Due to its unique application this therapy has several advantages over many other treatments and techniques.
- No medium (outside substance) is required unless a massage oil is used
- Can be applied over clothing
- Ideal for shy, nervous clients
- Ideal for the elderly, arthritic or disabled person
- Versatile
- Economical

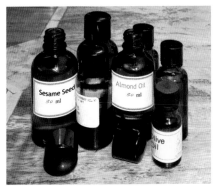

Although massage oil can be used to prolong the effect of treatment, one of the advantages of Indian head massage is that it can be applied almost anywhere, without any mediums.

- Minimal space is required.

These factors make Indian head massage an ideal therapy to use within the following:

- A general introduction to massage
- In the workplace
- Nursing/residential care
- As part of a stress management programme
- Demonstration at work.

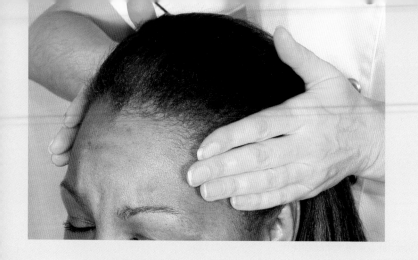

5 What To Expect From A Treatment

A fully qualified therapist who has been taught by a reputable institution should carry out the treatment. Very often the therapist will have a diploma on show.

A full Indian head massage treatment should include the following:

- An initial medical consultation, to discover any reason why the treatment should be adapted or if it is necessary to obtain a GP's permission. This can take anything up to half an hour.

- A complete treatment, starting from the back, neck, shoulders, scalp, face and ears. (Unless an adaptation is required following the initial consultation.)

- A continued consultation after the treatment, providing the client with after-care advice and a full explanation of any adverse reactions.

In addition to the above, the therapist must outline the full benefits of the treatment and explain the procedure, gaining

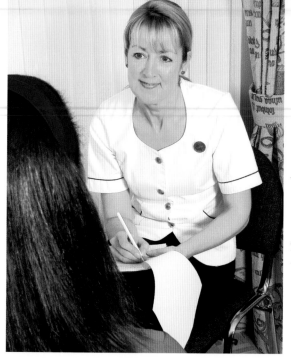

Be prepared to spend up to an hour and a half of your time at the initial consultation. An experienced practitioner will want to compile a detailed medical history in order to provide you with the best possible treatment.

the client's approval to carry out the treatment.

This whole process may take up to an hour and a half, depending on the depth of consultation and treatment applied. If the therapist feels adaptation is necessary, then the timing of the treatment will vary. The oil scalp massage will probably be shorter due to the vigorous techniques applied.

AFTER-CARE ADVICE

Aftercare is an important part of any treatment, encouraging the client to have a more holistic approach to their lifestyle. It is therefore important that the client follows a home-care programme in between treatments.

After-care also helps to prolong treatment, and, by following the after-care tips, the beneficial effects of each treatment can last up to a week!

24 HOURS AFTER TREATMENT

- Avoid (or a least cut down as much as possible)

41

stimulants such as tea, coffee, alcohol and cigarettes.

- Increase water intake, preferably up to two litres (three-and-a-half pints) per day. Try to drink still water rather than carbonated.
- Eat a light diet of fresh fruit, salad, and vegetables. Avoid red meat, dairy products and spicy foods.
- Practise breathing exercises to encourage relaxation.
- Encourage yourself to take regular relaxation periods.
- Take regular exercise.

LONG-TERM AFTER-CARE

An Indian head massage practitioner aims to improve your general health by reducing stress levels. Therefore, it is important to take advice for the longer term.

This may involve some elements included in short-term after-care (such as regular exercise), as well as:

- Practising self-massage
- Practising relaxation techniques, such as yoga, visualisation or meditation
- Continuing with

complementary therapies, such as Indian head massage, aromatherapy, and reflexology.

A FINAL NOTE
Remember that prevention is better than cure! If you can identify trigger factors for ill-health – such as stress and poor diet – addressing these issues at an earlier stage, and seeking the means to resolve them, can only be beneficial to your health.

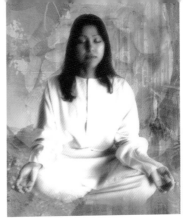

Relaxation techniques, such as meditation, help to prolong the effects of treatment as well as improve your general health and reduce your stress levels.

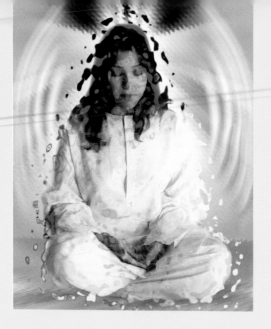

6 Words Of Warning

The process and techniques used in Indian head massage are part of an ongoing detoxifying programme. This means that the massage will encourage toxins to the skin's surface while the body is balancing and harmonising itself.

Indian head massage is a very safe and effective therapy, but much depends on the therapist and their training.

To date, no major side effects of the therapy have been reported. This is thought to be due largely to the professional manner in which the courses have been developed. Considered medical advice and guidance have been incorporated into such teaching schemes.

CONTRA-INDICATIONS

As with any form of massage, there are the usual contra-indications to be observed.

As well as observing the prospective client for any immediate obvious contra-

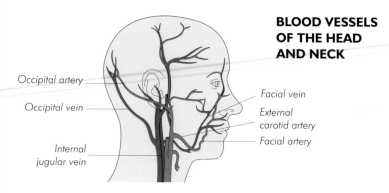

BLOOD VESSELS OF THE HEAD AND NECK

Occipital artery

Occipital vein

Internal jugular vein

Facial vein

External carotid artery

Facial artery

It is vital that the therapist is aware of any medical conditions that may affect the application of head massage. For example, blood clots and narrowed arteries should not be treated with massage.

indication, practitioners should also ensure that they *never* treat the following conditions:

- Thrombosis or embolism. Treatment may be given once the clot has dissolved.

- Cancer of the blood.
- Infectious diseases. Once recovery has commenced, treatment may be given.
- Septic conditions.
- Surgery. If surgery is less than six months old and above shoulder level, Indian head massage should not be applied.
- Pregnancy, if the woman is considered to be at risk or unstable. A normal pregnancy can be treated very lightly, after the first term.
- High temperature, illness or fever.
- Infectious diseases.
- Skin infections or inflammation, etc.
- Localised dilation of blood vessels, such as Aneurosa (commonly the artery in the temple/forehead area within the elderly).
- Intoxication.

CONDITIONS REQUIRING CAUTION

In addition to conditions that should not be treated with Indian head massage, there are a number of disorders that require the massage to be applied with caution, i.e. gently. These include:

- Osteoporosis. This is not totally contra-indicated. The treatment would need to be adapted using relaxing movements, rather than stimulating ones.
- Frailty. Relaxed movements only should be used.
- Chronic fatigue. Again, relaxing movements only should be used.
- Spondylitis or spondylosis in the neck. Again, use gentle movements only.
- Painful cysts. Treatments must be as gentle as possible.
- Psoriasis. This condition is not contagious, but caution needs to be taken.

ADVERSE REACTIONS

Sometimes, there may be possible adverse side-effects following treatment. While these are unusual, it is wise to be aware of them. Most clients give positive feedback, but occasional adverse reactions include:

- **Aching:** Because Indian head massage changes the

individual's posture, the affected muscles may have relaxed in a different position from before, which can cause aching.

- **Extreme tiredness:** Following treatment, the body is in a comfortable state of relaxation; in some cases, this can leave the client feeling very tired.
- **Heightened emotional state:** Indian head massage promotes physical, psychological and emotional well-being (see page 14). Following treatment, these elements can be so in-tuned with each other that the individual may feel a heightened emotional state.

If an adverse reaction should occur, you must remember that Indian head massage treatment is about releasing stress, tension and emotional imbalance. Explain to your therapist how you feel. He or she will be able to make modifications to their techniques, as well as suggesting methods to improve after-care.

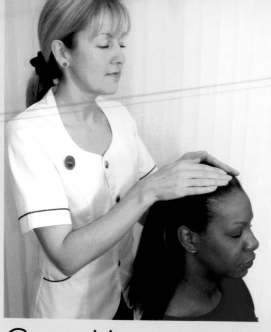

7

Case Histories

The following case histories have been included to illustrate how Indian head massage can be used to treat a range of problems.

❶ NECK ACHE

THE CLIENT
SW is a 44-year-old teacher.

THE PROBLEM
Five years ago, SW was involved in a car accident, in which she sustained neck injuries. Since then, she has suffered severe neck ache, leading to intensive headaches.

SW was taking medication for inflammation of the muscles, and painkillers for headaches. Her symptoms were ongoing, occurring at least three times a week.

SW found that her neck ache meant she was averaging only four to five hours of sleep per night, and, as a result, tension was building up in her back muscles.

TREATMENT

SW had a course of Indian head massage treatment over a six-week period. Now she claims to be sleeping – on average – seven hours per night.

The inflammation in her neck has decreased, due to having less tension in the back and neck muscles. On average, she has decreased her use of painkillers by 50 per cent.

SW says she feels better in her self and can focus on her family and future without enduring constant pain.

CLIENT'S COMMENTS

"Unbelievable! I could never imagine that something so gentle could have such a warm and calming effect. I would recommend this treatment to anyone – no harm could possibly come of it!"

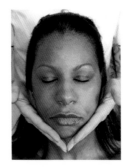

Neck pain and insomnia are just two problems that can be helped with Indian head massage.

❷ PARKINSON'S DISEASE

THE CLIENT
PF is a 59-year-old woman, retired due to disability.

THE PROBLEM
PF was diagnosed with Parkinson's disease two years ago, after suffering a family bereavement.

Since her diagnosis, PF has been taking medication for her condition. Unfortunately, this has had side-effects, for which she is taking additional medication.

PF's family describe her as once being a chatty and lively person. Unfortunately, her personal loss meant she was suffering mentally, physically and emotionally.

TREATMENT
PF's consultant suggested Indian head massage for relaxation and calmness within, hoping that this would help to slow the disease progression.

PF's progress under a course of head massage was

53

amazing. While she was undergoing a treatment, her shaking slowed – a fact that was noted both by herself and by her therapist.

Following treatment, PF now feels hopeful about life again, and is at a stage where she is beginning to believe in herself.

CLIENT'S COMMENTS
"I came to Indian head massage because I was desperate for something to help me. It was like being somewhere else other than this world. Indian head massage is my sanctuary and I shall continue to have treatment."

❸ THYROID PROBLEMS

THE CLIENT
AR is a 26-year-old social welfare officer, described as young and dynamic.

THE PROBLEM
AR had her thyroid removed two years ago, and has been on thyroxin medication since.

AR was suffering from extreme mood changes, and was feeling very discontented with her life in general.

In addition, AR complained of pain in her lower back, which she suggested was due to working on a computer for long periods of time.

TREATMENT
AR was looking for alternative ways to make her feel less discontented with life.

After four treatments, AR feels at peace and she is clear and positive about her future.

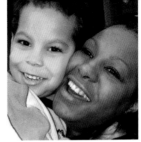

Indian head massage aims to heal the mind as well as the body, promoting harmony in our daily lives.

CLIENT'S COMMENTS
"It's the colours that really made me appreciate that the therapy was working. Where they came from I do not know, but they certainly left me feeling calmer and happier within myself."

❹ CONSTIPATION

THE CLIENT
CK is a 36-year-old solicitor.

THE PROBLEM
CK had terrible constipation, for which she was taking prescribed medication. CK also complained of severe stress, consuming above-average levels of alcohol to combat this.

TREATMENT
I believed CK's constipation was linked to stress. She seemed to be constantly 'on the go', six days a week, with only snippets of time to eat.

After two treatments, we discussed a time-management plan, creating time for rest and relaxation. As a result, CK is not as constipated!

CLIENT'S COMMENTS
"Who would have thought the simplicity of relaxation would have such an effect physically and psychologically. It has made me appreciate my life and everything in it."

❺ PSORIASIS

THE CLIENT
RB is an 18-year-old student.

THE PROBLEM
RB suffered from psoriasis, mainly on the back of the neck.

TREATMENT
RB's lifestyle was somewhat typical of a teenager – late nights, pubs and clubs. However, she spent a great deal of time worrying about her life, which caused her stress. All of this was aggravating her skin condition.

After six treatments, which encouraged deep relaxation, RB now worries less and concentrates on her life here and now.

CLIENT'S COMMENTS
"Wow, these treatments are amazing! My mum asked me to try them out and it's like being in another world. My friends have noticed the difference in me and my skin condition is not as angry."

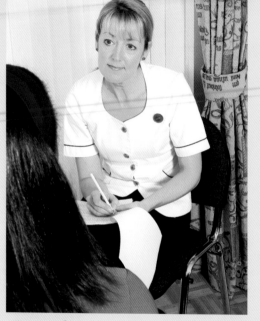

8

Finding A Practitioner

Indian Head Massage has become increasingly popular in the West, with an increasing number of people choosing to train in the therapy.

Courses are now run by examining boards nationwide, and it is advised that anyone seeking to try out this treatment asks to see their potential therapist's qualifications.

Although there are several courses available in head massage, the author practises the technique laid down by the Confederation of Ayurdevic Therapists (CAT) and the Confederation of Indian Head Massage (CIHM).

LEARNING MORE

If you are interested in learning the art of Indian head massage to practise yourself, contacts for courses run by CAT/CIHM are given at the end of this chapter.

Courses are run throughout the UK and are delivered by the author, a recognised expert in this field.

COURSE CONTENT
- An authentic approach to Indian head massage, investigating the spiritual and healing aspects of the therapy.
- A look at the key features that can be applied to Indian head massage, e.g. colour therapy, sound/music therapy, chakra balancing and consultation guide.
- A comprehensive look at the authentic techniques covering the back, neck, shoulders, head, face and ears.
- An additional oil scalp massage.
- A flexible course that contains both taught and self-directed learning aspects to enable students to complete the diploma at their own pace and at their convenience.

CAUTION!
Please note: not all therapies are the same. Techniques will vary depending on your tutor's guidance and training.

CAT/CIHM does not hold any responsibilities to any

other courses taught that bear the same title of Indian head massage.

The Indian head massage that is explained here in *Understanding Indian Head Massage*, and in *Authentic Indian Head Massage 'Malish'*, refers to a unique concept with a philosophy and practical technique taught only by Kush Kumar on behalf of the Confederation of Indian Head Massage.

CONTACTS
For information about CIHM and details of courses available, contact CIHM or Kush Kumar.

WEBSITE
www.cihm.org

EMAIL
kkumar@ayurvedictherapy.f9.co.uk

TELEPHONE
07703 263132

About the author

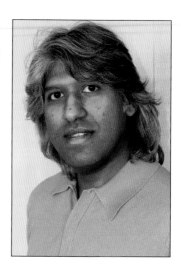

Kush Kumar is a fully qualified lecturer, therapist and author. He was brought up with Indian head massage and has travelled extensively to enhance his knowledge.

Kush founded the Confederation of Indian Head Massage, and also teaches for the Confederation of Ayurvedic Therapy.

In addition to *Understanding Indian Head Massage*, Kush's other books include *Authentic Indian Head Massage 'Malish'*, and the recently written *National Curriculum for Indian Head Massage* (for Edexel).

ACKNOWLEDGEMENTS
Special thanks to Dave Oldridge for photography (www.dopix.co.uk).

Other titles in the series

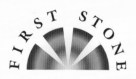

First published in 2004 by First Stone Publishing
PO Box 8, Lydney, Gloucestershire, GL15 6YD

The contents of this book are for information only and are not intended as a substitute for appropriate medical attention. The author and publishers admit no liability for any consequences arising from following any advice contained within this book. If you have any concerns about your health or medication, always consult your doctor.

ISBN 1 904439 29 2

Printed and bound in Hong Kong through Printworks International Ltd.